The Science of Bedtime Weight

A Closer Look at Evening Changes

Dr. James Rim

Table of contents

Chapter 1

Introduction

The Concept Of Weight Fluctuations Between Dinner And Bedtime

The concept of weight fluctuations between dinner and bedtime is a fascinating and intricate phenomenon that occurs within the human body during the evening hours. While our weight may appear to be relatively constant throughout the day, closer observation reveals that it can subtly shift during this specific time frame. This phenomenon is influenced by a combination of factors, including digestion, metabolism, hormones, and dietary choices. Let's explore the key aspects of this concept:

1. *Digestive Processes:* After consuming a meal, the digestive system initiates a complex process of breaking down food into its constituent nutrients. As the body

extracts essential nutrients like carbohydrates, proteins, and fats, it also absorbs water. The act of digestion and absorption leads to changes in the body's overall weight, particularly if the meal is substantial.

2. *Nutrient Utilization:* The body utilizes the nutrients obtained from the evening meal for various functions, including energy production, cell repair, and maintenance. Depending on the types and quantities of nutrients

consumed, the body's utilization processes can contribute to fluctuations in weight. For example, carbohydrates are converted into glucose, which is either used immediately for energy or stored as glycogen for later use. Glycogen is bound to water molecules, leading to temporary weight increases.

3. *Water Retention:* The consumption of certain foods, especially those high in sodium, can lead to water retention. The body holds onto water

to maintain fluid balance, which can result in an increase in weight. Additionally, as the body breaks down carbohydrates and stores them as glycogen, water molecules are bound to glycogen molecules, contributing to water retention and weight fluctuations.

4. *Hormonal Influences:* Hormones play a significant role in regulating various bodily functions, including metabolism, appetite, and fluid balance. Hormones like insulin,

cortisol, and even melatonin (which regulates sleep) can influence how the body manages nutrients and fluids. Hormonal fluctuations that occur during the evening can impact weight changes.

5. *Time of Day and Activity Levels:* The time of day and your level of physical activity can also affect weight fluctuations. As the day progresses, your activity levels might decrease, causing fewer calories to be burned. This can impact how your body

processes and stores nutrients, potentially leading to weight changes. Additionally, your body's metabolism tends to slow down as you prepare to sleep, which can influence how nutrients are utilized and stored.

6. *Psychological Factors:* Emotional and psychological factors, such as stress, relaxation, and mood, can also play a role in evening weight fluctuations. Emotional eating or consumption of comfort foods in the evening may contribute to weight

changes. Moreover, stress can impact hormone levels, affecting how the body processes and stores nutrients.

Understanding the concept of weight fluctuations between dinner and bedtime involves recognizing the intricate interplay of digestion, nutrient utilization, hormones, and lifestyle factors. While these fluctuations may seem minor, they provide insights into how our bodies respond to the daily rhythms of nourishment, metabolism, and rest.

By delving into this concept, we gain a deeper appreciation for the complexity of our physiological processes and how they influence our overall well-being.

The Significance Of Understanding These Changes For Overall Health And Wellness.

Understanding the changes in weight that occur between dinner and bedtime holds significant implications for overall health and wellness. While these fluctuations might seem minor or even inconsequential, they offer valuable insights into the intricate workings of our bodies and can guide us toward making informed choices that positively impact our well-being. Here's why understanding these changes is so important:

1. *Insight into Metabolic Health*: The shifts in weight during the evening hours provide a window into our metabolic processes. By observing

how our bodies respond to different foods and the timing of meals, we can gain insights into our metabolism's efficiency. Recognizing how specific foods and habits influence weight changes allows us to tailor our diet and lifestyle choices to support optimal metabolic health.

2. Hormonal Balance and Regulation: Hormones play a central role in weight regulation and overall health. Understanding how hormones like insulin, cortisol, and melatonin interact during the evening hours can provide insights into our body's hormone balance. This knowledge empowers us to make choices that support hormonal harmony, which in turn can contribute to improved weight management and well-being.

3. *Prevention of Overeating and Mindful Eating:* Being aware of the potential for weight fluctuations in the evening can help us make mindful choices about our eating habits. Recognizing that the body's

response to certain foods might lead to temporary weight increases encourages us to practice moderation and mindfulness when consuming meals and snacks. This awareness can prevent overeating and promote a healthier relationship with food.

4. *Informed Dietary Choices:* Understanding how different nutrients are processed by the body in the evening hours allows us to make more informed dietary choices. For example, knowing how

carbohydrates and sodium affect water retention can influence our decisions about the types and amounts of food we consume in the evening. This knowledge can support healthier eating patterns and weight management.

5. *Personalized Lifestyle Modifications*: No two individuals are exactly alike, and our bodies respond differently to various factors. By understanding the changes that occur between dinner and bedtime,

we can tailor our lifestyle choices to our unique needs. This might involve adjusting meal timing, considering the types of foods we consume, and aligning our habits with our body's natural rhythms.

6. *Empowerment and Active Health Management:* Knowledge is power, and understanding the science behind evening weight changes empowers us to take an active role in our health management. Rather than feeling at the mercy of fluctuations on

the scale, we can approach our well-being with a sense of agency. Armed with insights, we can make proactive choices that align with our health goals.

7. *Holistic Approach to Wellness:* Our overall health is a holistic tapestry woven from various factors—nutrition, exercise, sleep, stress management, and more. Recognizing the significance of evening weight changes contributes to a more comprehensive understanding of

wellness. It encourages us to view health as an interconnected journey and motivates us to adopt habits that support our well-being on multiple levels.

In essence, comprehending the changes in weight that occur between dinner and bedtime goes beyond a mere fascination with numbers. It invites us to explore the intricate dance of our body's responses, encouraging us to make thoughtful choices that harmonize with our physiology. By embracing this knowledge, we empower ourselves to embark on a journey of well-informed decisions, holistic health, and a deeper connection to our bodies' intricate mechanisms.

Chapter 2

The Dinner Effect: Exploring Immediate Weight Shifts

The Impact Of A Meal On Body Weight

The impact of a meal on body weight is a dynamic and multifaceted phenomenon that involves various physiological processes within the body. When you consume a meal, whether it's a light snack or a substantial dinner, several factors come into play that can lead to changes in your body weight. Here's a closer look at the impact of a meal on body weight:

1. *Food Consumption:* When you eat a meal, you're introducing a combination of macronutrients (carbohydrates, proteins, and fats) and micronutrients (vitamins and minerals) into your body. The total caloric content of the meal, as well as the types of nutrients present, can

influence the immediate impact on your body weight.

2. Digestion and Nutrient Absorption: Digestion is the process through which your body breaks down the food you've consumed into its basic components—nutrients that can be absorbed and used by your cells. This process involves enzymes and gastric acids that break down complex molecules into simpler forms for absorption. As digestion progresses, nutrients are absorbed through the walls of your stomach and intestines into your bloodstream.

3. *Water Retention:* The consumption of food can trigger temporary shifts in your body's water balance. Some nutrients, like sodium, can influence fluid retention, leading to a temporary increase in body weight due to water weight. Additionally, carbohydrates are stored in your body as glycogen, which binds to water molecules. Consuming carbohydrates can lead to

an increase in glycogen stores and water retention.

4. *Nutrient Utilization:* Once absorbed, nutrients are transported to various cells throughout your body to provide energy, support growth, and maintain bodily functions. Carbohydrates are converted into glucose, which fuels your brain and muscles. Fats are utilized for energy and cell membrane structure, while proteins are broken down into amino acids for cellular repair and growth.

5. *Thermogenesis:* The process of digestion and nutrient utilization requires energy, known as the thermic effect of food (TEF). TEF contributes to the number of calories your body burns while processing and utilizing the nutrients from your meal. While the impact of TEF on overall body weight is relatively small, it's an example of how your body expends energy to process food.

6. *Hormonal Responses:* Eating triggers hormonal responses that

regulate various aspects of digestion, metabolism, and energy balance. Hormones like insulin, which helps regulate blood sugar levels, play a role in nutrient uptake and utilization. Hormones also influence hunger and satiety cues, which can impact future eating behaviors and meal frequency.

7. *Individual Variation:* It's important to note that the impact of a meal on body weight can vary greatly from person to person. Factors such as metabolism, genetics, age, activity

level, and overall health can influence how your body responds to food intake. Some individuals may experience more noticeable fluctuations in weight after a meal, while others might see minimal changes.

In essence, the impact of a meal on body weight is a combination of nutrient intake, digestion, nutrient absorption, water retention, nutrient utilization, energy expenditure, and hormonal responses. While immediate weight fluctuations after a meal are often temporary, long-term patterns of food consumption and lifestyle choices play a more significant role in overall weight management and health. Understanding how these factors interact can empower you to make informed choices about your diet and lifestyle.

Digestion, Nutrient Absorption, and Water Retention: Contributions to Short-Term Weight Changes

The human body is a marvel of complexity, and nowhere is this more evident than in the intricate dance of digestion, nutrient absorption, and water retention. These processes interweave in a symphony that can lead to short-term weight changes after a meal. Let's explore how each element contributes to this phenomenon:

1. *Digestion:* Digestion is the process by which the body breaks down the food you eat into its component nutrients. This process begins in the mouth with chewing and the release of enzymes, and continues in the stomach and intestines. As food is broken down into smaller particles, it becomes more accessible for nutrient extraction.

2. *Nutrient Absorption:* Once food is broken down, the nutrients within

it—such as carbohydrates, proteins, fats, vitamins, and minerals—are absorbed through the walls of the stomach and intestines and into the bloodstream. The bloodstream then transports these nutrients to cells throughout the body, where they are used for energy production, growth, repair, and other vital functions.

3. *Water Retention:* Water retention is a process in which the body temporarily holds onto water due to various factors, including the

consumption of certain foods and minerals. Sodium, for instance, plays a significant role in fluid balance. Consuming foods high in sodium can lead to fluid retention, resulting in a temporary increase in weight. Similarly, carbohydrates are stored in the body as glycogen, and each molecule of glycogen binds to water molecules. The storage of glycogen can lead to increased water weight.

4. Short-Term Weight Changes: The combined effects of digestion, nutrient absorption, and water retention can result in short-term weight changes. Here's how it works:

- Digestion: As you eat, your stomach and intestines fill with food and fluids. This added weight contributes to an immediate increase in the scale reading. However, this weight is not indicative of fat gain; it's a temporary reflection of the volume of food and fluids you've consumed.

- Nutrient Absorption: As nutrients are absorbed into the bloodstream, they are transported to cells throughout your body. This process can lead to an increase in overall body weight due to the addition of nutrients being carried by the bloodstream.

- Water Retention: The consumption of sodium-rich foods, along with carbohydrate intake that leads to glycogen storage, can both contribute to water retention. This retained water adds to your body's weight in the short term.

It's important to note that these short-term weight changes are primarily due to variations in water content, nutrient absorption, and food volume. They are not reflective of significant changes in body fat. These fluctuations are a normal part of the body's physiological processes and should not be cause for concern.

In essence, the interplay of digestion, nutrient absorption, and water retention can lead to short-term weight changes after a meal. These fluctuations are largely related to changes in water content, nutrient distribution, and the volume of food consumed. Understanding these processes can help you interpret weight changes with a more informed perspective, recognizing that they are a natural part of how your body responds to nourishment.

How Different Types Of Meals Can Lead To Varying Weight Shifts

The type of meal you consume can have a significant impact on the short-term weight shifts you might experience. Different nutrients and food components interact with your body in unique ways, influencing factors such as digestion, nutrient absorption, and water retention. Here's how various types of meals can lead to varying weight shifts:

1. *Carbohydrate-Rich Meals:* Meals that are rich in carbohydrates, such as pasta, rice, bread, and starchy vegetables, can lead to noticeable short-term weight shifts. Carbohydrates are stored in the body as glycogen, which binds to water molecules. For every gram of glycogen stored, the body retains several grams of water. Therefore, consuming a carbohydrate-heavy meal can lead to an increase in water

retention, resulting in a temporary weight increase.

2. *High-Sodium Meals:* Foods high in sodium, such as processed foods, restaurant dishes, and certain condiments, can contribute to water retention. Sodium plays a role in regulating fluid balance in the body, and consuming excess sodium can lead to increased water retention. This can result in a short-term increase in weight due to the retained fluids.

3. Protein-Rich Meals: Protein-rich meals, like those containing lean meats, poultry, fish, eggs, and plant-based protein sources, can have a different effect on weight shifts. Protein is essential for tissue repair and growth. While protein itself doesn't lead to water retention to the same extent as carbohydrates, the process of digestion and nutrient utilization requires energy, contributing to the thermic effect of food (TEF). TEF leads to a small increase in energy expenditure and could impact short-term weight shifts.

4. *Balanced Meals with Fiber:* Meals that include a balanced combination of carbohydrates, proteins, healthy fats, and fiber-rich foods (like fruits, vegetables, and whole grains) can contribute to a more stable weight response. Fiber, in particular, can promote feelings of fullness and reduce the rapid spikes in blood sugar that can occur after consuming

high-sugar or high-carbohydrate meals.

5. *Fluid Intake:* Fluid intake also plays a role in short-term weight shifts. If you consume a large amount of fluids with your meal, you might experience temporary weight changes due to the added volume of liquids in your stomach. This effect is particularly evident if you consume beverages that are high in calories or sodium.

6. *Nutrient Density:* The nutrient density of your meal, or the concentration of vitamins, minerals, and other essential nutrients per calorie, can also influence weight shifts. Meals that are rich in nutrients can support overall health and potentially have a positive impact on your body's responses to food.

7. *Individual Variability:* It's important to note that individual responses to different types of meals can vary based on factors such as metabolism,

genetics, activity level, and overall health. Some individuals may be more sensitive to water retention from carbohydrates or sodium, while others may experience minimal changes.

In summary, the composition of your meal—whether it's carbohydrate-rich, high in sodium, protein-rich, balanced, or fluid-heavy—can influence short-term weight shifts. Understanding how various nutrients interact with your body's processes can help you interpret weight changes more accurately and make informed dietary choices that align with your health and wellness goals.

Chapter 3

Metabolism at Twilight: Unraveling
Evening Processes

The Body's Metabolism During The Evening Hours

As the sun sets and the day transitions into evening, your body's metabolism undergoes a subtle shift. Metabolism, the complex set of processes that convert food into energy and fuel various bodily functions, doesn't remain constant throughout the day. Instead, it follows a rhythmic pattern influenced by your body's internal clock, known as the circadian rhythm. Here's a closer look at how your metabolism operates during the evening hours:

1. *Slower Metabolic Rate:* As evening approaches, your body's metabolic rate tends to slow down. This phenomenon is in part influenced by your body's natural circadian rhythm, which prepares you for rest and sleep. The decrease in metabolic rate means

that your body requires fewer calories to maintain its functions compared to the more active daytime hours.

2. *Energy Conservation:* During the evening, your body shifts its focus from energy expenditure to energy conservation. This is especially true if you're not engaging in vigorous physical activity. Your body recognizes the impending period of rest and prioritizes the preservation of energy resources for essential functions like cell repair, immune system

maintenance, and brain activity during sleep.

3. Nutrient Utilization and Storage: During the evening hours, your body continues to utilize nutrients from the meals you've consumed throughout the day. Carbohydrates that were converted into glucose are used to provide energy for various bodily functions. Excess glucose may be stored in the liver as glycogen, while any surplus calories from fats and proteins might be stored as body fat.

4. *Hormonal Influences:* Hormones play a significant role in regulating metabolism and energy balance. During the evening hours, hormone levels shift to reflect your body's readiness for rest. For example, melatonin—a hormone that promotes sleep—is released, leading to a decrease in alertness and physical activity. The hormone leptin, which regulates appetite, may also influence how hungry you feel during this time.

5. Impact of Evening Meals: The meals you consume during the evening hours can impact your metabolism. While your metabolic rate naturally slows down in the evening, consuming a large and calorie-dense meal can lead to increased energy intake. Since your body's energy expenditure is lower during this time, excess calories from a late and heavy dinner may contribute to weight gain over time.

6. Maintaining a Healthy Routine: While your metabolism does slow down in the evening, it's essential to focus on maintaining a healthy routine that aligns with your body's natural rhythms. Opt for balanced and nutrient-dense meals during the evening hours. Avoid consuming large amounts of high-calorie, high-sugar, or high-sodium foods, as these can have a more significant impact on your body's metabolism during this period.

The Role Of Hormones Such As Insulin, Cortisol, And Melatonin In Weight Regulation

Hormones act as powerful messengers within the body, influencing various physiological processes, including weight regulation. Insulin, cortisol, and melatonin are three key hormones that play distinct roles in maintaining a balance between energy intake, expenditure, and overall health. Here's a closer look at how these hormones impact weight regulation:

1. Insulin:

Role: Insulin is a hormone produced by the pancreas that plays a central role in regulating blood sugar levels and nutrient utilization. When you eat carbs, your body converts them to glucose, which is then absorbed into the circulation. In reaction, the pancreas secretes insulin to aid in the movement of blood glucose into cells for use as fuel or storage.

Impact on Weight Regulation:

- Blood Sugar Control: Insulin helps regulate blood sugar levels by facilitating the uptake of glucose into cells. This prevents blood sugar from rising to dangerous levels after meals.

- Fat Storage: Insulin also promotes the storage of excess glucose as glycogen in the liver and muscles. Once these storage spaces are full, extra glucose is converted to fat and stored in adipose tissue.

- Appetite Regulation: Insulin can influence appetite and satiety. Rapid fluctuations in blood sugar levels, often triggered by consuming sugary or refined carbohydrate-rich foods, can lead to hunger and overeating.

2. Cortisol:

Role: Cortisol is a stress hormone produced by the adrenal glands. It plays a crucial role in the body's stress response and helps regulate metabolism, immune function, and blood sugar levels.

Impact on Weight Regulation:
- Metabolism and Fat Storage: Cortisol can influence metabolism and energy

expenditure. In times of stress, cortisol prompts the body to use stored glucose for immediate energy. Additionally, cortisol can stimulate the breakdown of fats and proteins for energy.

- Abdominal Fat Accumulation: Chronic stress and elevated cortisol levels have been associated with an increased tendency to accumulate fat, particularly around the abdominal area.

- Appetite and Cravings: Cortisol can affect appetite and food preferences.

Some individuals may experience increased cravings for high-calorie, comfort foods during periods of stress.

3. Melatonin:

Role: Melatonin is a hormone produced by the pineal gland, primarily at night, and it plays a key role in regulating sleep-wake cycles (circadian rhythms).

Impact on Weight Regulation:

- Sleep Regulation: Melatonin helps regulate sleep patterns by signaling to the body that it's time to rest. Maintaining a healthy weight requires getting enough sleep.

- Metabolism: Disruption of the natural circadian rhythm due to irregular sleep patterns or exposure to artificial light at night can impact metabolism and potentially lead to weight gain.

- Appetite Regulation: Melatonin can influence appetite and eating behavior. Some research suggests that sleep deprivation and circadian rhythm disturbances can lead to altered appetite hormones and increased food intake.

How Metabolism Differs During Restful Periods Versus Activity

Metabolism is a dynamic process that adapts to the body's energy needs. It varies based on different factors, including the state of restfulness or activity. Here's a comparison of how metabolism differs during restful periods and activity:

1. Restful Periods:

During restful periods, such as when you're sleeping or at rest without engaging in physical activity, your metabolism undergoes specific changes:

- Basal Metabolic Rate (BMR): BMR represents the number of calories your body needs to maintain basic functions at rest. It includes the energy required for essential processes like breathing, maintaining body temperature, circulating blood, and supporting organ function. BMR accounts for the largest portion of your daily energy expenditure, even when you're not physically active.

- Lower Energy Expenditure: Since your body is at rest, your energy expenditure is generally lower compared to when you're active. This is because fewer calories are needed for muscle contractions, movement, and other physical activities.

- Fat Utilization: During rest, your body primarily relies on stored fat as a source of energy. This is especially true during periods of extended fasting, such as overnight during sleep.

- Tissue Repair and Growth: Restful periods are crucial for tissue repair, cell renewal, and growth. Hormones released during sleep, like growth hormone, support these processes.

2. Activity:

When you engage in physical activity, your metabolism shifts to accommodate the increased energy demands:

- Increased Energy Expenditure: Physical activity requires energy, and the intensity and duration of the activity determine how much energy is expended. Movement, muscle contractions, and exercise-related processes contribute to a higher calorie burn.

- Elevated Heart Rate: Physical activity increases heart rate and breathing rate, which are essential for delivering oxygen and nutrients to muscles and other tissues. This increased demand on the cardiovascular system contributes to higher energy expenditure.

- Carbohydrate Utilization: During moderate to intense activity, the body primarily uses carbohydrates as a source of quick energy. Glucose stored as glycogen in the muscles and liver is converted into energy to fuel physical exertion.

- Afterburn Effect: After intense activity, the body continues to expend more energy than usual, a phenomenon known as excess post-exercise oxygen consumption (EPOC) or the "afterburn" effect. This is due to the need to restore energy stores and repair muscle tissue.

- Muscle Development: Engaging in resistance or strength training during activity can lead to muscle building and development. Muscle tissue has a higher metabolic rate than fat tissue, so increased muscle mass contributes to a higher resting metabolic rate.

Chapter 4

Nighttime Nutrient Utilization:
Fueling The Body As You Sleep

How The Body Uses Stored Nutrients During Sleep

Sleep is a critical period for your body to rest, repair, and restore itself. While you're asleep, various physiological processes continue to operate, including the utilization of stored nutrients to support essential functions. Here's how the body uses stored nutrients during sleep:

1. Glycogen Stores: Glycogen is the storage form of glucose (sugar) that is primarily stored in the liver and muscles. During sleep, your body taps into its glycogen stores to provide a steady supply of glucose to maintain normal blood sugar levels and ensure that essential bodily functions continue. This process helps prevent low blood sugar (hypoglycemia) while you're fasting during the night.

2. Energy Supply for Basic Functions: Even during restful sleep, your body requires energy to support essential functions such as breathing, circulating blood, and maintaining body temperature. Stored nutrients, particularly glucose derived from glycogen, are used to provide the necessary energy for these basic physiological processes.

3. Protein Synthesis and Repair: While you sleep, your body is actively

engaged in protein synthesis and repair. This is when tissues are repaired, muscle fibers are regenerated, and cellular maintenance occurs. Amino acids, the building blocks of proteins, play a crucial role in this process. These amino acids can come from protein sources you've consumed throughout the day and those derived from the breakdown of proteins in your body.

4. Hormone Regulation: Sleep is a time when hormonal processes are at

work, including the release of growth hormone. Growth hormone plays a vital role in tissue repair, cell regeneration, and growth. During sleep, the body uses amino acids to support the synthesis of new proteins and the repair of damaged tissues.

5. Fat Utilization: During sleep, your body's reliance on glucose as an energy source decreases. Instead, your body shifts toward using stored fats as an energy source, particularly during periods of extended fasting

such as overnight. This process is crucial for maintaining energy levels and preserving glucose for essential functions.

6. Brain Function: Even as you sleep, your brain remains active and requires energy to support vital functions like maintaining cognitive processes, regulating body temperature, and orchestrating neural signaling. Stored nutrients, especially glucose, are used to fuel these ongoing brain activities.

7. Supporting Immune Function:
Sleep is also a time when your immune system works to defend your body against pathogens and repair damaged cells. Nutrients obtained from your diet and stored nutrients are utilized to support immune function and promote overall health.

8. Hormonal Balance:
Sleep plays a role in regulating hormones that impact appetite, metabolism, and energy balance.

Hormones like leptin and ghrelin, which influence hunger and satiety, are regulated during sleep. Adequate sleep helps maintain hormonal balance, supporting healthy eating habits and weight management.

The Dynamic Duo: The Role Of Glycogen And Fat Utilization For Energy

Within the intricate workings of the human body lies a fascinating energy management system—a delicate balance between the utilization of two key fuel sources: glycogen and fat. These energy powerhouses play distinct roles in providing the fuel needed to support various physiological activities. Let's unravel the roles of glycogen and fat utilization for energy, exploring how they contribute to your daily vitality.

Glycogen: The Instant Energy Reservoir

Glycogen takes center stage as the body's immediate energy reserve—a quick-release fuel source readily available to meet the demands of sudden activity. Primarily stored in the liver and muscles, glycogen is derived from glucose, the simple sugar obtained from carbohydrates in your diet. Here's how glycogen contributes to your energy needs:

1. Quick Burst of Energy: When you engage in activities requiring rapid bursts of energy—whether it's a sprint, a weightlifting set, or a sudden burst of movement—glycogen comes to the rescue. It provides a quick and easily accessible source of glucose that can be rapidly converted into energy, allowing you to perform at your best in high-intensity situations.

2. Supporting Brain Function: The brain relies heavily on glucose for energy, and glycogen plays a critical

role in maintaining stable blood sugar levels to nourish brain cells. This is particularly crucial during situations of increased mental focus and concentration.

3. Preventing Hypoglycemia: Glycogen serves as a buffer against low blood sugar levels (hypoglycemia). During periods of fasting or extended periods between meals, your body can tap into glycogen stores to release glucose into the bloodstream, ensuring that

your brain and other vital organs receive a steady supply of energy.

Fat Utilization: The Endurance Dynamo

While glycogen provides quick bursts of energy, stored fats are the endurance champions that fuel your body during longer, sustained activities. Fats are stored in adipose tissue throughout the body, and they become a reliable energy source when glycogen levels are depleted.

Here's how fat utilization supports your energy needs:

1. Sustained Energy: When you engage in low to moderate-intensity activities—such as jogging, cycling, or prolonged walking—your body shifts to utilizing stored fats as a primary energy source. Fats are broken down into fatty acids and transported to muscles, where they are oxidized to produce energy.

2. Endurance Activities: During activities that extend beyond a quick burst, such as long-distance running or endurance training, fat utilization becomes increasingly important. Fat stores offer a virtually endless supply of energy, making them ideal for activities that require prolonged effort.

3. Energy Storage and Insulation: Fats also play a role in energy storage, serving as a repository for excess calories consumed in your diet.

Additionally, adipose tissue serves as insulation, helping to regulate body temperature and protect internal organs.

The Harmonious Balance: Adaptation and Utilization

Your body is a master of adaptation, seamlessly switching between glycogen and fat utilization based on the energy demands of the moment. The balance between these two fuel sources is not fixed; it adapts to your activity level, dietary intake, and individual physiology. During rest and light activities, fats dominate as the primary energy source. As the intensity of your activities increases, glycogen takes center stage to provide the quick energy needed for explosive movements.

Timing Your Meals: Unveiling The Impact On Nighttime Nutrient Utilization

Meal timing isn't just about satisfying your hunger—it can significantly influence how your body utilizes nutrients during the crucial hours of rest. As the day transitions into night and you prepare to lay down for sleep, the choices you make about when to eat can have a notable impact on nighttime nutrient utilization. Let's delve into this intricate dance between meal timing and your body's nighttime processes.

1. Evening Meal Composition: The composition of your evening meal plays a pivotal role in how your body

manages nutrients during sleep. Opting for a balanced meal that includes complex carbohydrates, lean proteins, healthy fats, and fiber can provide a steady supply of nutrients throughout the night.

- Complex Carbohydrates: Incorporating complex carbohydrates, like whole grains, vegetables, and legumes, provides a sustained release of glucose into the bloodstream. This gradual release helps maintain stable blood sugar levels, preventing drastic spikes and crashes that could disrupt sleep.

- Proteins: Consuming lean proteins supports muscle repair and growth during the night. Amino acids derived from proteins contribute to cellular regeneration and tissue maintenance, ensuring that your body thrives even as you slumber.

- Healthy Fats: Including sources of healthy fats, such as avocados, nuts, and seeds, contributes to satiety and provides a source of sustained energy. Fats also aid in the absorption of fat-soluble vitamins.

- Fiber: Foods rich in fiber promote digestive health and a feeling of fullness. This can be especially beneficial to prevent discomfort or hunger pangs during the night.

2. Blood Sugar Regulation: Eating meals high in refined sugars or simple carbohydrates before bedtime can lead to rapid spikes and crashes in

blood sugar levels. These fluctuations not only disturb your sleep but can also impact your body's nighttime nutrient utilization.

- Insulin Sensitivity: Consuming excessive sugar or refined carbohydrates can lead to an overproduction of insulin, potentially affecting your body's insulin sensitivity over time. This may impact your ability to regulate blood sugar effectively during sleep.

3. Meal Timing and Digestion: Your body's digestive system operates at a somewhat slower pace during sleep. Consuming heavy, large meals close to bedtime can lead to discomfort and disrupted sleep due to increased digestive activity. It's advisable to allow ample time between your last meal and bedtime to ensure proper digestion.

4. Late-Night Snacking: Late-night snacking, especially on calorie-dense and high-sugar foods, can impact

your body's nutrient utilization during sleep. Consuming excess calories late at night may lead to increased fat storage due to reduced energy expenditure during sleep.

5. Impact on Hormones: Meal timing can influence the release of hormones such as insulin, which plays a role in blood sugar regulation. Eating balanced meals at appropriate times helps maintain hormonal balance and supports energy regulation.

Chapter 5

Harmony in the Night: Exploring the Intricate Balance of Hormones Involved in Weight Regulation During Sleep

While the world slumbers, your body orchestrates a symphony of hormonal activity that influences weight regulation, metabolism, and overall well-being. The delicate balance of hormones during sleep is a marvel of biological choreography, impacting everything from appetite to energy expenditure. Let's delve into the complex interplay of these hormones and their role in guiding your body's nighttime journey toward optimal weight regulation.

1. Leptin: The Satiety Sentinel

Role: Leptin, often referred to as the "satiety hormone," is secreted by fat cells and signals to your brain that you're full and satisfied after eating.

Impact During Sleep: During the night, leptin levels continue to rise and fall in response to your body's energy status. Adequate sleep is essential for maintaining optimal leptin levels. Sleep deprivation can lead to reduced leptin levels, causing your brain to perceive a state of hunger and prompting increased food intake.

2. Ghrelin: The Hunger Herald

Role: Ghrelin, the "hunger hormone," is secreted primarily by the stomach and signals your brain when it's time to eat.

Impact During Sleep: Sleep deprivation can lead to increased ghrelin levels, resulting in heightened feelings of hunger. This hormonal imbalance can trigger overeating and disrupt your body's natural hunger and satiety cues.

3. Insulin: The Blood Sugar Regulator

Role: Insulin plays a crucial role in regulating blood sugar levels by facilitating the uptake of glucose into cells.

Impact During Sleep: Stable blood sugar levels during sleep are essential for overall well-being. Consuming high-sugar or high-carbohydrate foods close to bedtime can lead to rapid spikes and crashes in blood sugar levels, impacting insulin sensitivity and potentially contributing to weight gain over time.

4. Growth Hormone: The Tissue Regenerator

Role: Growth hormone is released in pulses during deep sleep and supports tissue repair, cellular regeneration, and muscle growth.

Impact During Sleep: Adequate sleep is necessary for the proper release of growth hormone. This hormone promotes the maintenance and growth of lean body mass, which in turn contributes to a higher resting metabolic rate and enhanced weight regulation.

5. Cortisol: The Stress Responder

Role: Cortisol, often dubbed the "stress hormone," is released by the adrenal glands in response to stress and helps regulate metabolism and blood sugar levels.

Impact During Sleep: Cortisol levels should naturally decrease during the evening to promote relaxation and sleep. Disrupted sleep patterns or high-stress levels can lead to elevated cortisol levels at night, impacting sleep quality and potentially influencing weight gain.

6. Melatonin: The Sleep Regulator

Role: Melatonin, the "sleep hormone," is secreted by the pineal gland in response to darkness and helps regulate the sleep-wake cycle.

Impact During Sleep: Melatonin not only promotes restful sleep but also plays a role in metabolism regulation. Disrupted sleep patterns or exposure to artificial light at night can affect melatonin production and potentially impact weight regulation.

Hormonal Choreography: How Changes Influence Appetite And Metabolism

Behind the scenes of your daily life, a remarkable hormonal dance is constantly unfolding, shaping your appetite and metabolism. These intricate hormonal changes are not only essential for maintaining energy balance but also play a significant role in your body's weight regulation. Let's delve into this choreography and understand how hormonal shifts influence your appetite and metabolism.

1. Leptin: The Satiety Conductor

Role: Leptin, produced by fat cells, is often referred to as the "satiety hormone." It signals to your brain that you're full and satisfied after eating.

Impact on Appetite and Metabolism: Adequate leptin levels help regulate your appetite. When you've eaten enough, leptin is released, and your brain receives the message that you're no longer hungry. However, chronic overeating or obesity can lead to a condition known as leptin resistance, where the brain becomes less responsive to leptin's signals, leading to persistent feelings of hunger.

2. Ghrelin: The Hunger Messenger

Role: Ghrelin, secreted mainly by the stomach, is the "hunger hormone." It stimulates appetite and promotes food intake.

Impact on Appetite and Metabolism: Ghrelin levels increase before meals and decrease after eating. This hormone initiates the sensation of hunger and motivates you to seek food. During weight loss efforts, ghrelin levels can increase, potentially leading to heightened hunger and making it more challenging to maintain a calorie deficit.

3. Insulin: The Blood Sugar Regulator

Role: Insulin is a hormone that helps regulate blood sugar levels by facilitating glucose uptake into cells.

Impact on Appetite and Metabolism: Insulin plays a role in appetite regulation by influencing how the body uses and stores energy. After a meal, insulin levels rise to help cells absorb glucose for energy. Consuming high-sugar or high-carbohydrate foods can lead to rapid spikes in insulin levels, followed by crashes that trigger hunger and cravings.

4. Cortisol: The Stress Modulator

Role: Cortisol, produced by the adrenal glands, helps regulate metabolism and responds to stress.

Impact on Appetite and Metabolism: Stress-induced cortisol release can impact appetite and metabolism.

While acute stress might temporarily reduce appetite, chronic stress can lead to overeating and weight gain. Elevated cortisol levels may influence fat storage, particularly in the abdominal region.

5. Thyroid Hormones: The Metabolic Maestros

Role: Thyroid hormones (T3 and T4) regulate metabolism by influencing how cells use energy.

Impact on Appetite and Metabolism: Optimal thyroid function is crucial for maintaining a healthy metabolism. An underactive thyroid (hypothyroidism) can lead to a slower metabolism and weight gain, while an overactive thyroid (hyperthyroidism) can increase metabolism and appetite.

6. Peptide YY (PYY) and Cholecystokinin (CCK): The Satiety Supporters

Role: PYY and CCK are hormones released in response to food intake, signaling fullness.

Impact on Appetite and Metabolism: PYY and CCK contribute to feelings of satiety after eating. They help control the pace of digestion, ensuring that nutrients are absorbed gradually, which can help regulate blood sugar levels and prevent rapid spikes and crashes that lead to hunger.

Untangling the Web: Disrupted Sleep's Impact on Hormonal Balance and Weight

Sleep isn't just a period of rest—it's a critical physiological process that impacts every aspect of your well-being, including hormonal balance and weight regulation. Disrupted sleep can throw these delicate systems into disarray, setting the stage for a cascade of effects that can influence your appetite, metabolism, and ultimately, your weight. Let's delve into the potential implications of disrupted sleep on hormonal balance and weight.

1. Leptin and Ghrelin Dysregulation:

Sleep deprivation can lead to alterations in the levels of leptin and ghrelin—the dynamic duo that regulates appetite. Leptin levels decrease, making your brain less responsive to signals of fullness, while ghrelin levels increase, boosting feelings of hunger. This hormonal imbalance can lead to overeating and weight gain.

2. Insulin Sensitivity Disruption:

Disrupted sleep can impair insulin sensitivity, leading to higher insulin levels. Elevated insulin levels promote fat storage and make it more challenging for your body to utilize stored fat for energy. Over time, this can contribute to weight gain and an increased risk of type 2 diabetes.

3. Cortisol and Stress Response:

Sleep deprivation triggers an increase in cortisol levels, mimicking the body's stress response. Elevated cortisol can lead to increased fat storage, particularly around the abdominal region. This can result in "stress-related weight gain," as chronic sleep disruption perpetuates this hormonal cycle.

4. Appetite for High-Calorie Foods:

Disrupted sleep can lead to altered food preferences, with a heightened desire for calorie-dense and sugary foods. The hormonal shifts caused by sleep deprivation can increase cravings for comfort foods, potentially leading to overconsumption and weight gain.

5. Increased Caloric Intake: Sleep-deprived individuals often consume more calories overall. This can be attributed to hormonal changes that amplify appetite and cravings, coupled with impaired decision-making and self-control due to fatigue.

6. Impaired Energy Balance

The combination of increased caloric intake and decreased physical activity due to fatigue can lead to a disrupted energy balance. This imbalance can contribute to weight gain over time.

7. Metabolic Slowdown:

Sleep deprivation can slow down metabolism. A sluggish metabolism makes it harder for your body to burn calories efficiently, making weight management more challenging.

8. Circadian Rhythm Disruption:

Disrupted sleep patterns can disrupt your body's natural circadian rhythms. This can lead to irregular hormone secretion, including melatonin and growth hormone, which play roles in sleep quality and weight regulation.

Chapter 6

Unveiling the Impact: How Physical Activity Affects Evening Weight Changes

Physical activity isn't just a daytime pursuit—it has a profound influence on your body's dynamics even as the evening approaches. The choices you make regarding exercise can set the stage for weight changes and metabolic shifts that extend into the evening hours. Let's explore how physical activity impacts weight changes in the evening and beyond.

1. Boosting Caloric Expenditure: Engaging in physical activity throughout the day can increase your total daily energy expenditure. This means you burn more calories not only during exercise but also afterward, leading to a potential reduction in overall caloric intake.

2. Afterburn Effect (Excess Post-Exercise Oxygen Consumption - EPOC): After engaging in moderate to intense physical activity, your body's metabolism remains elevated for a period after the exercise session. This "afterburn" effect results in continued calorie burning even as you rest, contributing to the overall energy deficit for the day.

3. Muscle Activation and Metabolism: Physical activity, particularly resistance training or strength exercises, stimulates muscle activation and growth. Muscle tissue has a higher resting metabolic rate compared to fat tissue, which means that having more muscle can lead to a higher baseline calorie burn, even at rest.

4. Appetite Regulation: Physical activity can impact appetite regulation. While intense exercise can initially suppress appetite, prolonged or high-intensity activity might lead to increased hunger later in the day. The timing and intensity of your physical activity can influence your appetite cues in the evening.

5. Metabolic Rate Elevation: Regular physical activity increases your basal metabolic rate (BMR), which is the number of calories your body burns at rest. This elevated BMR persists even as you transition into the evening hours, contributing to increased energy expenditure throughout the day.

6. Insulin Sensitivity Improvement: Physical activity improves insulin sensitivity, making your body more efficient at using glucose for energy. This can help regulate blood sugar levels and prevent spikes that could lead to fat storage.

7. Fat Oxidation: Depending on the intensity and duration of your physical activity, your body may switch to utilizing stored fat as an energy source. This can contribute to overall fat loss and improved body composition.

8. Psychological Impact: Engaging in physical activity can positively impact your mood and stress levels. Reduced stress and improved mood can potentially prevent emotional eating in the evening, leading to healthier food choices.

Embrace the Twilight Move: Benefits of Light Exercise Before Bedtime

When the day winds down and the evening beckons, engaging in light exercise might be the perfect way to bid farewell to the day and prepare your body for restful slumber. While intense workouts close to bedtime may disrupt sleep, gentle and mindful movement offers a host of benefits that can enhance your overall well-being. Let's explore the advantages of incorporating light exercise into your evening routine before bedtime.

1. Stress Reduction: Light exercise, such as gentle stretching or yoga, can help alleviate stress and tension accumulated throughout the day. Mindful movement encourages relaxation, allowing you to unwind and transition from the hustle of the day to a peaceful state of mind.

2. Improved Sleep Quality: Engaging in light exercise can promote better sleep quality. Activities like gentle stretching or restorative yoga can relax your muscles and ease your body into a state of relaxation, making it easier to fall asleep and enjoy uninterrupted sleep.

3. Enhanced Blood Circulation: Light exercise encourages blood circulation, which can help deliver oxygen and nutrients to your body's tissues. This gentle boost in circulation can provide a sense of vitality and relaxation, contributing to an overall sense of well-being.

4. Mood Enhancement: Movement triggers the release of endorphins, the "feel-good" hormones. Engaging in light exercise can lift your spirits, reduce anxiety, and create a positive mindset that carries into the evening and your sleep.

5. Flexibility and Mobility:
Incorporating gentle stretches or mobility exercises can enhance your flexibility and joint range of motion. Improved flexibility not only supports better movement throughout the day but also helps prevent stiffness upon waking.

6. Calming the Mind: Light exercise, such as deep breathing or meditation, can help calm the mind and create a sense of mindfulness. This relaxation can counter the stresses of the day and set the stage for a peaceful night's rest.

7. Heart Health: Light exercises, such as a leisurely walk, can contribute to cardiovascular health by promoting blood flow, regulating blood pressure, and supporting overall heart function.

8. Digestive Aid: Gentle movement can aid digestion by promoting the movement of food through your digestive tract. This can help prevent discomfort or indigestion that might disrupt your sleep.

9. Establishing Routine: Incorporating light exercise into your evening routine creates a ritual that signals your body that it's time to wind down. This consistent routine can help regulate your body's internal clock and improve sleep patterns.

Balancing Act: Potential Impact of Intense Exercise on Sleep Quality and Weight

While exercise is a cornerstone of a healthy lifestyle, the timing and intensity of your workouts can have a profound impact on both your sleep quality and weight management. Intense exercise is a double-edged sword that can yield positive results for fitness while also potentially affecting sleep and weight. Let's explore the potential impact of intense exercise on sleep quality and weight and how to strike a balance for optimal well-being.

1.   Positive   Impact   on   Sleep: Engaging in regular, intense exercise can promote better sleep quality over time. When done earlier in the day, intense exercise can help regulate your body's internal clock, leading to improved sleep patterns and deeper sleep stages.

2. Adverse Impact on Sleep: Intense exercise close to bedtime may disrupt sleep quality. High-intensity workouts elevate heart rate, body temperature, and adrenaline levels, making it harder for your body to transition into a state of relaxation conducive to sleep.

3. Hormonal Influence: Intense exercise releases endorphins and stimulates the production of cortisol, which can elevate stress levels. Exercising too close to bedtime can lead to increased cortisol levels at a time when they should naturally be decreasing, potentially affecting sleep.

4. Recovery and Muscle Repair: Intense exercise places stress on muscles and tissues. Adequate recovery is crucial for muscle repair and growth. Poor recovery due to disrupted sleep can hinder muscle recovery and overall performance.

5. Weight Management: Intense exercise can contribute to weight loss by burning calories and increasing metabolic rate. However, if your exercise regimen is extremely intense and unsustainable, it might lead to overcompensation through increased appetite and potential overeating.

6. Hunger and Cravings: Intense exercise can increase hunger and cravings, especially if not followed by proper refueling. This could potentially lead to consuming excess calories and hindering weight management efforts.

7. Balancing Energy Expenditure and Intake: If your intense exercise leads to a substantial increase in calorie expenditure, there's a risk of compensatory eating. Overestimating calorie burn and underestimating food intake can impede weight loss.

8. Timing Matters: The timing of intense exercise can determine its impact on sleep and weight. Engaging in high-intensity workouts during the morning or early afternoon may have positive effects on sleep, while nighttime workouts might disrupt sleep patterns.

Chapter 7

Unraveling the Mind-Plate Connection: Psychological Factors Influencing Evening Eating Behaviors

Eating behaviors aren't solely governed by physical cues; the intricate interplay between your mind and your plate is a crucial factor in determining your dietary choices, particularly in the evening. A combination of emotions, habits, and psychological factors can lead to specific eating behaviors during this time. Let's delve into some of the psychological factors that contribute to eating behaviors in the evening.

1. **Emotional Eating:** Emotional triggers, such as stress, boredom, loneliness, or anxiety, can prompt eating in the evening. Food often becomes a way to cope with emotions, leading to mindless snacking or overeating.

2. **Reward and Pleasure**: The evening might be perceived as a time to

unwind and treat oneself. Food, particularly indulgent or comfort foods, can be associated with reward and pleasure, leading to cravings for these foods during the evening.

3. Habitual Patterns: Evening eating behaviors can become habitual over time. For instance, if you're accustomed to having a snack while watching TV or surfing the internet in the evening, these routines can trigger automatic eating even if you're not truly hungry.

4. Availability and Accessibility: The presence of food and its accessibility can influence eating behaviors. If unhealthy snacks are readily available in the evening, you might be more likely to consume them, even if you're not particularly hungry.

5. Social Influence: Social interactions and gatherings in the evening can influence eating behaviors. Eating can be a social activity, and the desire to fit in or share a meal with others can lead to eating more than intended.

6. Mindful vs. Mindless Eating: Mindless eating—consuming food without paying attention to hunger or fullness cues—can be a result of multitasking, distraction, or eating while engaged in other activities. Mindful eating, on the other hand, involves being present and fully experiencing the sensory aspects of eating.

7. Cravings and Triggers: Evening can be a time when specific cravings emerge. The sight, smell, or even thought of certain foods can trigger intense desires, leading to consumption even if you're not actually hungry.

8. Deprivation and Restriction: Restrictive diets or calorie deprivation during the day can lead to increased hunger and cravings in the evening. This can result in overeating or consuming energy-dense foods in the evening.

9. Perceived Stress and Control: Stress might make people eat emotionally or turn to food for solace. Additionally, the evening might provide a sense of control, and some individuals may restrict their intake throughout the day only to overindulge in the evening.

Chapter 8

Navigating the Twilight Zone: Lifestyle Choices and Their Impact on Evening Weight Changes

The choices you make throughout the day extend their influence well into the evening, and this includes lifestyle habits such as alcohol consumption and caffeine intake. These choices can play a pivotal role in your evening weight changes, impacting your sleep, metabolism, and overall well-being. Let's explore how alcohol consumption and caffeine intake can influence your evenings and the weight changes that might result.

1. Alcohol Consumption:

Impact on Evening Weight:
Alcohol is a source of empty calories that can contribute to weight gain if consumed in excess. Consuming alcohol in the evening can lead to an increase in calorie intake, potentially

disrupting the balance between energy expenditure and intake.

Impact on Sleep Quality:
While alcohol might initially induce drowsiness, it can disrupt sleep patterns and impair the quality of your sleep. This can lead to inadequate rest, which in turn affects metabolism, hunger hormones, and weight management.

Impact on Appetite Regulation:
Alcohol consumption can influence appetite regulation by affecting hormone levels, including ghrelin and leptin. This disruption in appetite cues might lead to overeating or consuming calorie-dense foods in the evening.

2. Caffeine Intake:

Impact on Evening Weight:
Caffeine is a stimulant that can boost metabolism and temporarily suppress

appetite. However, consuming caffeine too close to bedtime might disrupt sleep and affect overall weight management.

Impact on Sleep Quality:
Caffeine is known to interfere with sleep quality and disrupt the natural sleep-wake cycle. Consuming caffeine in the afternoon or evening can delay the onset of sleep, leading to less restful sleep and potential weight-related consequences.

Impact on Stress and Hormones:
Excessive caffeine intake can lead to increased stress levels and the release of cortisol, which can influence appetite and fat storage. Evening emotional eating might be caused by high levels of stress.

3. Hydration and Fluid Balance:

Impact on Evening Weight:
Alcohol and caffeine are diuretics, meaning they can increase urine output and contribute to fluid loss.

This can lead to temporary weight fluctuations due to changes in fluid balance.

Impact on Sleep Quality:
Dehydration caused by alcohol and caffeine consumption can impact sleep quality and lead to nighttime awakenings. Adequate hydration is important for overall well-being and restful sleep.

Water—the elixir of life—plays a crucial role in maintaining your body's equilibrium and supporting various physiological functions. Hydration isn't just about quenching your thirst; it's about nourishing your cells, regulating bodily processes, and even influencing water retention. Let's delve into the importance of hydration and how it affects water retention.

1. Cellular Function:

Importance of Hydration:
Hydration is essential for optimal cellular function. Water is the medium in which biochemical reactions occur, facilitating nutrient transport, waste removal, and cellular communication.

Effect on Water Retention:
Proper hydration helps maintain a healthy fluid balance within cells. When you're adequately hydrated, cells are less likely to retain excess water, preventing the bloated feeling associated with water retention.

2. Electrolyte Balance:

Importance of Hydration:
Electrolytes like sodium, potassium, and magnesium help regulate fluid balance and nerve function.

Maintaining the right balance is crucial for proper muscle contractions and overall homeostasis.

Effect on Water Retention:
Adequate hydration supports electrolyte balance, preventing imbalances that can lead to water retention. Proper levels of electrolytes ensure that water is distributed effectively throughout the body's compartments.

3. Kidney Function:

Importance of Hydration:
The kidneys play a pivotal role in filtering waste and excess fluids from the bloodstream. Hydration supports efficient kidney function, allowing for the elimination of waste products and excess fluids.

Effect on Water Retention:
When you're hydrated, your kidneys can effectively eliminate excess sodium and water through urine.

Dehydration, on the other hand, can lead to kidney dysfunction and potential water retention.

4. Hormone Regulation:

Importance of Hydration:
Hydration is vital for hormonal balance. Hormones like vasopressin regulate water excretion, ensuring that your body maintains the right level of hydration.

Effect on Water Retention:

Adequate hydration supports the regulation of vasopressin, preventing excessive water retention. When you're dehydrated, vasopressin levels may increase, leading to water retention.

5. Digestive Health:

Importance of Hydration:

Water aids in digestion by supporting the movement of food through the gastrointestinal tract and promoting the breakdown of nutrients.

Effect on Water Retention:
Proper hydration can prevent constipation and bloating, which are often associated with water retention in the gastrointestinal tract.

Strategizing Success: Practical Tips for Optimizing Lifestyle Choices for Weight Regulation

Embarking on a journey to support weight regulation requires a holistic approach that encompasses your daily lifestyle choices. By making mindful decisions in various areas of your life, you can create a supportive environment that fosters balance, health, and well-being. Here are some practical tips to help you optimize your lifestyle choices for effective weight regulation:

1. Prioritize Balanced Nutrition:

- Embrace whole, nutrient-dense foods rich in fiber, lean proteins, healthy fats, and a variety of vitamins and minerals.
- Opt for balanced meals that include a mix of carbohydrates, proteins, and fats to promote satiety and stabilize blood sugar levels.

- Practice portion control to avoid overeating and mindless snacking.

2. Hydration Matters:

- Aim to drink water consistently throughout the day to support proper hydration.
- Choose water over sugary drinks or excessive caffeine to prevent dehydration and its potential impact on cravings.

3. Mindful Eating:

- Pay attention to hunger and fullness cues, and eat slowly to allow your body to register satiety.
- Minimize distractions while eating to fully savor your meals and prevent overconsumption.

4. Regular Physical Activity:

- Incorporate a mix of cardiovascular exercise, strength training, and flexibility work into your routine.

- Find activities you enjoy to promote consistency and make exercise a part of your daily life.

5. Quality Sleep:

- Make sleep a priority by creating a sleep-friendly atmosphere and a regular sleep routine.
- To assist hormone regulation and general wellbeing, aim for 7-9 hours of restful sleep each night.

6. Stress Management:

- Engage in relaxation techniques such as deep breathing, meditation, yoga, or hobbies you enjoy.
- Take care of yourself to reduce stress and avoid emotional eating and cortisol-related weight gain.

7. Balanced Meal Timing:

- To avoid acute hunger and overeating in the evening, aim for frequent and balanced meals throughout the day.

- Avoid large meals close to bedtime to promote digestion and a comfortable night's sleep.

8. Mindset and Attitude:

- Cultivate a positive relationship with food, exercise, and your body. Avoid negative self-talk or unrealistic expectations.
- Focus on health and well-being rather than solely on weight loss.

9. Limit Alcohol and Caffeine Intake:

- Drink alcohol sparingly and keep in mind that it contains calories.
- Limit caffeine intake, especially in the afternoon and evening, to support sleep quality.

10. Plan and Prepare:

- Plan your meals and snacks ahead of time to avoid last-minute unhealthy choices.

- Keep wholesome snacks on hand to avoid reaching for less wholesome ones.

11. Seek Support:

- Enlist the help of a registered dietitian, personal trainer, or support group to provide guidance and accountability.

Weight regulation is a journey that involves a multitude of lifestyle choices working in harmony. By taking a holistic approach and implementing these practical tips, you're creating a foundation for sustainable, balanced, and positive change. Keep in mind that over time, little, regular measures can produce huge outcomes. Prioritize your well-being, listen to your body, and approach your goals with patience and self-compassion.

Chapter 9

Conclusion: Navigating the Path to Health and Balance

In the pages of "The Science of Bedtime Weight: A Closer Look at Evening Changes," we've embarked on a journey to uncover the intricate dance of our bodies between dinner and bedtime. As we wrap up this exploration, let's reflect on the lessons we've learned and the path we've walked.

From understanding the dynamic shifts in weight due to digestion, nutrient absorption, and hydration, to delving into the role of hormones, metabolism, and lifestyle choices, we've gained a comprehensive understanding of how our bodies respond during the evening hours. Armed with this knowledge, we're equipped to make informed choices that contribute to our well-being and weight management.

In a world where health and balance are often sought after, our journey reminds us that success is found in the small steps—the daily decisions that align with our goals and aspirations. As we stand at this conclusion, let's carry these key principles forward:

1. Mindful Awareness:
- Knowledge empowers change. Becoming aware of how our bodies

respond in the evening enables us to make mindful choices that nurture our health.

2. Holistic Balance:
- Striking a balance in our evening routines, from nutrition to relaxation, is a cornerstone of both weight management and overall well-being.

3. Customization and Progress:
- Every journey is unique. Personalizing our choices to fit our

lifestyles and celebrating the progress we make reinforces positive habits.

4. Patience and Resilience:
- Sustainable change takes time. Embracing patience and maintaining resilience in the face of challenges are key to long-term success.

5. Positive Intent:
- Approach each evening with positivity. Embrace the opportunity to

care for yourself and make choices that support your health and happiness.

With the closing of this chapter, our journey continues. Armed with newfound insights, we navigate our evenings with a deeper understanding of our bodies and a commitment to nurturing our well-being. Here's to a future filled with balanced choices, vibrant health, and the joy of living in harmony with ourselves.